Ketogenic Diet Fat Bombs

50+ Irresistible Sweet and Savory Recipes for Weight Loss that Everyone Can Enjoy

By Jennifer Sullivan

Table of Contents

Introduction

I want to thank you and congratulate you for joining me in my book, *Ketogenic Diet Fat Bombs: 50+ Irresistible Sweet and Savory Recipes for Weight Loss that Everyone Can Enjoy*.

The Ketogenic Diet is one that is taking the world by storm. It gets its name from 'ketogenesis' which is a process where the body starts to burn fat for energy instead of carbohydrates. When the right balance is achieved with your diet, the liver starts to produce ketones. These ketones are made from fat and they can then be used as fuel for the body and the mind.

The key markers of a ketogenic diet are high fat intake and low carbohydrate intake. People on this diet should also try to eat a moderate amount of protein with each meal.

The Ketogenic Diet is used for many to help them reach their weight loss goals. For others, it is used to manage conditions like diabetes and frequent seizures. Regardless, some people choose to test their ketone levels. This is especially important for diabetics following the diet, since the production of too many ketones can lead to a condition called ketoacidosis.

The good news is that boring food is not on the menu for the Ketogenic diet. You also do not have to give up desserts, which is what this book will be about. Between the pages of this book, you will find dozens of sweet or savory desserts to enjoy on the Ketogenic Diet. You will find cakes, bars, candy, frozen treats, and more. These 'fat bombs' are incredibly tasty and the best part is that you can eat them without guilt.

Grab a few sticky notes! You are definitely going to want to try out some of these desserts for later.

Section I:
Candy and Fudge

Butter Pecan White Chocolate Fat Bombs

Who doesn't love sweet and creamy white chocolate? These fat bombs will melt in your mouth and they have plenty of butter pecan flavor. The best part? They have less than 1 carb per serving but all the flavor of a dessert packed full of sugar.

Ingredients

- 2 ounces cocoa butter

- ½ cup pecans (chopped)

- 2 tablespoons butter

- 2 tablespoons coconut oil

- 2 tablespoons powdered sugar substitute of your choice

- ¼ teaspoon vanilla extract

- 1/8 teaspoon liquid artificial sweetener of choice

- 1/8 teaspoon salt

Instructions

Add the cocoa butter, butter, and coconut oil to a small pan and warm them over medium heat until they have all melted. Turn off the stove and add the powdered sweetener to the melted butters. Then, stir in the salt. Next, stir in the liquid sweetener and the vanilla extract.

Butter Pecan White Chocolate Fat Bombs

Once all the ingredients are well-combined, set the mixture to the side for a moment. Distribute the chopped pecans among candy molds or silicone mini cupcake molds. Then, pour in the white chocolate mixture and transfer to the freezer immediately. Freeze for 30 minutes before enjoying and store in the freezer. These will melt very easily, though this makes for a pleasant eating experience.

Salted Coconut Almond Bark

Who doesn't love salt and chocolate? This sweet-and-salty pair is one that can only be made better with the sweetened taste from coconut and the crunch from wholesome almonds. You can break this bark into 12 pieces and enjoy it for less than 4 grams of net carbs.

Ingredients

- ½ cup coconut butter

- ½ cup unsweetened coconut flakes

- ½ cup almonds

- 2 cups (100 grams) 80-90% dark chocolate

- 10 drops liquid sweetener (optional and to taste)

- ½ teaspoon almond extract

- ¼ teaspoon coarse sea salt

Instructions

Start by setting the oven to 350 degrees so it can preheat. Line a baking sheet with foil and then spread the coconut and almonds across it. Place these in the oven to toast. This should take 5-8 minutes and you should stir every 3-4 minutes to prevent burning. Then, set this pan to the side so everything can cool.

Raspberry Cheesecake Truffles

Next, start warming the chocolate in a double boiler. Once most of it is melted, stir in the coconut butter and mix until smooth. Then, add the sweetener if you choose and the almond extract. Stir to incorporate thoroughly and set to the side while you prepare a pan.

Line a baking sheet with parchment paper and pour the dark chocolate mixture into it. Use a spatula to create an even layer. Then, evenly distribute the toasted coconut and almonds on top of the chocolate. Finish this with a sprinkling of the sea salt.

Place this in the fridge for at least an hour. Once it is set, you can slice it with a knife or break it into pieces.

Raspberry Cheesecake Truffles

The dreamy flavor of melt-in-your-mouth raspberry cheesecake can only be made better with chocolate. These truffles have a rich raspberry cheesecake filling and a chocolate outer coating. You can enjoy one of these truffles for less than 2 net carbs.

Ingredients

For the filling:

- 1 cup raspberries (frozen)

- 1 cup full-fat cream cheese (softened)

- ½ cup almond flour

- ¼ cup coconut flour

- 2 tablespoons powdered sugar substitute of your choice

- 1 teaspoon sugar-free vanilla extract

- Liquid artificial sweetener to taste

For the coating:

- 1.4 ounces cocoa butter

- 2.8 ounces 90% dark chocolate

Raspberry Cheesecake Truffles

Instructions

Add the raspberries, cream cheese, sugar substitute, and vanilla to a food processor and process until smooth. Then, add the flours and pulse just long enough to mix them into the raspberry mixture. Then, add 2 tablespoons of the mixture to an ice cube tray, cake pop molds, or other silicone molds. Place these in the freezer for 45 minutes to an hour to firm up before the next step.

When you are almost ready to coat the truffles, warm the cocoa butter and dark chocolate in a double boiler. Once they melt completely, turn off the stove and let the mixture cool slightly. You do not want it to solidify, but you also do not want it to be hot enough to melt the raspberry truffles while you are coating them. Before you get started with the coating, line a baking tray with parchment paper and set it to the side.

Use a fork or toothpick to pierce the truffles in turn. Coat them one at a time, holding the raspberry ball over the bowl of chocolate and spooning the chocolate on top of it. You will need to turn the ball to coat it completely. You can stop turning once the chocolate solidifies. Place the finished truffle on the prepared baking tray. Once you are done, return the truffles to the refrigerator for at least 15 minutes to set before enjoying.

Ginger Fat Bombs

Ginger is found at the heart of many savory recipes and this is no exception. These have a spicy bite from the ginger with a slightly sweet taste from the coconut. The high coconut oil content means that your body will be burning fat in no time at all.

Ingredients

- ¾ cup coconut butter (melted)

- ¾ cup coconut oil (melted)

- ¼ cup unsweetened shredded coconut

- 1 teaspoon ginger (more or less to taste)

- 1 teaspoon granulated sugar substitute of your choice

Instructions

Add all the ingredients to a bowl and mix. Add sugar and ginger until you get the taste you desire. Once they are well incorporated, pour the mixture into an ice cube tray or silicone mold. Place these in the refrigerator for 1-2 hours, until completely set. This recipe makes 10 fat bombs.

Coconut Oil Fat Bomb Candies

Coconut oil is high in all the right kinds of fat to kick start your liver into ketogenesis. They are melt-in-your-mouth delicious and are perfect for satisfying a candy bar craving. You should note that the coconut oil needs to be softened but not melted- otherwise your candies will be nearly impossible to shape. If you want, you can roll the balls in unsweetened shredded coconut or sprinkle the coconut on top before refrigeration. These have less than 3 carbs in two of the candies and this recipe makes 9 servings.

Ingredients

- 1 cup softened cold-pressed virgin coconut oil

- 1-2 tablespoons artificial granulated sweetener of your choice (to taste)

- 3 tablespoons unsweetened cocoa powder

- 2 tablespoons almond butter

- 1 teaspoon vanilla extract

- ½ teaspoon sea salt

- Shredded coconut (optional)

Instructions

Add all the ingredients (except shredded coconut) to a large bowl and mix until smooth. You can also beat or use a food processor if you do not want to mix by hand.

Next, line a baking sheet with parchment or wax paper. Use a tablespoon and drop 'balls' of the mixture onto the paper. If you are using shredded coconut, you could drop the balls into the coconut and then place on the parchment paper. Handle the fat bombs as little as possible, since your body temperature can make the coconut oil melt.

Once you have made all the coconut oil candies, place them in the refrigerator until they become solid. Then, you can transfer to a container for storage in the refrigerator so you can enjoy one whenever you would like.

Easy Peanut Butter Fudge

Since there are no-sugar-added alternatives for peanut butter, it is a popular Keto Diet ingredient because of its high fat and protein content. This recipe calls for peanut butter and a few other ingredients to make a delicious fudge.

Ingredients

- 1 cup coconut oil

- 1 cup no-sugar-added peanut butter

- ¼ cup vanilla almond milk (unsweetened)

- 2 teaspoons vanilla liquid artificial sweetener (or to taste)

Instructions

Place the coconut oil and peanut butter in a small pan on the stove and warm over low heat. Once they are blended together well, add the mixture to a blender. Then, add the remaining ingredients and blend until they are all thoroughly incorporated.

Set the blender to the side while you line a loaf pan with parchment paper. Be sure to leave some hanging over on the sides for easy removal of the fudge once it has set. Then, pour the peanut butter mixture into the pan. Refrigerate about 2 hours, until it has set. Use the parchment paper to lift the fudge up and cut into 12 pieces.

Caramel Nut Clusters

Who doesn't love gooey caramel when it is paired with crunchy nuts and creamy dark chocolate? These candies are even better because coarse sea salt lets them satisfy a sweet-and-salty combination that is reminiscent of chocolate covered pretzels. This recipe makes 9 candies.

Ingredients

For the base of the candy:

- 9 sugar-free caramel hard candies of your choosing

- 18 macadamia nuts

- 9 pecans

- 1 teaspoon coarse sea salt

For the chocolate ganache:

- 40 grams (about 1 lightly packed cup) 85% dark chocolate

- 2-3 tablespoons heavy cream

- ¼ teaspoon vanilla extract

Instructions

Start by preheating the oven to 320 degrees. Place aluminum foil across a baking tray and arrange the nuts on them, with 1 pecan and 2 macadamia nuts in each cluster. You may want to

Caramel Nut Clusters

crack the macadamia nuts in half so they lay flat and do not roll around.

Position one caramel candy on each of the nut clusters. Once the oven is preheated, carefully place the baking tray inside so that the clusters do not roll around. You will want to watch the candies closely, but they should take about 10 minutes. The caramel should be melted just enough that each nut is secured into the cluster and not so long that they turn into puddles. Remove the candies when this happens and allow them to cool.

While you are waiting for the caramel to cool down, prepare the ganache to go on top. Use a double boiler to warm the heavy cream until it is almost bubbling. Stir in the vanilla and then add the dark chocolate and let it melt, stirring frequently. Once smooth, pour the ganache over the cooled clusters and sprinkle the coarse sea salt on top. Refrigerate for an hour before eating these candies.

Peppermint Fat Bombs

The coconut oil in these bites will kick your body into ketosis overdrive and leave you feeling fuller for longer. These have a fresh, minty taste that will remind you of a peppermint candy and chocolate to satisfy your sweet tooth. This recipe makes 12 servings.

Ingredients

- 1 1/3 cups coconut oil (melted)

- 4 tablespoons unsweetened cocoa

- 2 tablespoons granulated sugar substitute of your choice (or to taste)

- ½ teaspoon peppermint extract

Instructions

Put the coconut oil in a bowl and add the peppermint extract and sweetener. Stir until all the ingredients are thoroughly incorporated. Place half of this mixture into a bowl and set to the side. Pour the other half inside of a silicon mold or ice cube tray.

Place the try in your fridge while you prepare the second layer so it can start to firm. Stir the cocoa into the reserved peppermint mixture and mix until well-combined. You can add more sweetener if needed. If the white layer has started to set, pour this on top of it and return to the fridge at least 1-2 hours, until completely firm.

Peanut Butter Buckeyes

This low-carb alternative to a holiday favorite that can be enjoyed year round comes packed with flavor for just 5 net carbs per serving. This Buckeye is a rich, chocolatey outer cover enveloping a creamy peanut butter center.

Ingredients

- 1 ½ cups powdered sugar substitute of your choice

- 1 cup peanut butter

- 6 ounces sugar-free chocolate

- 4 tablespoons butter (melted)

Instructions

Add the melted butter, peanut butter, and powdered sugar to a bowl and mix together to form a batter. If it is too runny and does not seem like it will form, place the mixture in the refrigerator for 30 minutes to set before preparing the balls.

When you are ready, use your hands or a small cookie scoop to roll your balls. Each peanut butter ball should be about 2 tablespoons of the mixture. Place these on a baking sheet that has been lined with parchment paper. Once you have no batter remaining, chill the balls for at least 30 minutes before continuing to the next step. They will need to be very cold to hold their shape as you coat them with chocolate.

Once the batter is chilled enough, add the chocolate to a small, deep bowl and place it in the microwave. Cook for 10-20 seconds at a time, stirring around to disperse between intervals. It is warmed enough once it will easily roll off the spoon. However, you do not want it so warm that it will not stick to your truffles.

Use a spoon to transfer one peanut butter truffle at a time to the bowl. Roll it around in the chocolate and use a toothpick or fork to lift it out. Hold it over the bowl for a few seconds, allowing the extra chocolate to drip back into the bowl. Then, place the coated truffle back on the baking sheet and repeat with the remaining Buckeyes. Once you are done, let the entire batch cool for at least an hour in the refrigerator before eating.

Fudgy Macadamia Fat Bombs

Five easy ingredients and a mold are all it takes to make these delicious fat bombs. This has a soft, fudge-like consistency and the combination of sweet macadamia nuts with rich chocolate is to die for. The best part is these will have your body burning fat in no time at all.

Ingredients

- 4 ounces macadamia nuts (chopped)

- 2 ounces cocoa butter

- ¼ cup heavy cream

- 2 tablespoons powdered sugar substitute of your choice

- 2 tablespoons unsweetened cocoa powder

Instructions

Use a double boiler to melt your cocoa butter. Once melted, stir in the cocoa powder and powdered sugar substitute. Mix well until the sugar and cocoa powder dissolve completely. Then, stir in the macadamia nuts until well incorporated.

Once everything is warm, pour in the heavy cream. Stir frequently and allow this to come back up to temperature. Pour into your choice of molds and allow to cool before placing in the fridge. Let them sit for 1-2 hours to set. Afterward, you can store at room temperature and they will have a consistency that is slightly softer than that of chocolate.

Homemade Chocolate Truffles

As you would expect, these chocolate truffles melt in your mouth. This recipe contains honey. Even though this is not always a low-carb sweetening option, it works with this recipe because the small amount is distributed through 12 truffles so each has 3 carbs per serving. You can use a sweetener if you choose, however.

Ingredients

- 5 ounces 85% dark chocolate

- ½ cup heavy cream

- 2 tablespoons honey

- 2 tablespoons butter

- 2 tablespoons raw cocoa powder

- ½ teaspoon cinnamon

- ½ teaspoon pure vanilla extract

- 1/8 teaspoon sea salt

Instructions

Add the heavy cream to a pan and warm it over low heat. Do not let it boil or it may scald, giving your truffles a burnt taste. As you are waiting, chop your chocolate into small pieces. Add the chocolate and butter to the pan and stir constantly, maintaining a low heat until it is all melted together. Remove

Homemade Chocolate Truffles

the pan from heat and stir in the honey, cinnamon, vanilla, and salt.

Place the chocolate mixture in the fridge for about an hour, until it cools and hardens. You will want to stir this periodically, as butter the butter tends to separate out of the mix when it cools. Once the mixture is hardened, scoop up a small amount of truffle batter and shape it into a ball. You should be able to make 12 that are about 1 ½ inches across.

Place the balls on a tray or plate that has been covered with parchment paper. Place them in the refrigerator for about 30 minutes. Then, add the cocoa powder to a bowl and place the truffles inside. Roll the truffles gently until they are coated evenly with the powder.

Peppermint Cheesecake Fudge

This creamy fudge has a hint of peppermint. They are perfect for the holidays, but will also satisfy your sweet tooth craving any time of year. You can top with candy canes if you choose. Since they have sugar, limit how much you use or choose a sugar-free version. This recipe makes 8 servings with less than 3 carbs each.

Ingredients

- 20 ounces cream cheese (softened)

- 1 ½ cups butter (softened)

- 1 ½ cups powdered sugar substitute of choice

- 2 ½ teaspoons peppermint extract

- Few drops red food coloring (optional)

- Crushed candy cane pieces (optional)

Instructions

Take an 8x8 baking dish or glass pan and line with parchment paper. Make sure there is a little extra hanging over the sides-it will help you easily remove the bars after they have set.

Then, combine all the ingredients except the food coloring and candy cane pieces in a large bowl. Beat with an electric mixer until smooth. Alternatively, you could combine them in a food processor. If you want a stronger peppermint taste, add a little more extract.

Peppermint Cheesecake Fudge

Next, pour the mixture into the pan. If you would like the fudge to have red swirls, place 3-5 drops on top and swirl with a toothpick or knife. If you are using the candy cane pieces, sprinkle them across the top.

Place the prepared fudge in the fridge for 1-2 hours. Then, use the 'handles' to lift the fudge from the dish. Cut and enjoy or store in an airtight container for later.

Section II:
Brownies, Cookies, and Bars

Pumpkin Crumble Bars

Pumpkin is definitely a fall favorite. These bars pair a pumpkin layer with a smooth and creamy texture with a heavenly coffee cake crumble on top. These are so good you may want to skip having them for dessert and just make them to enjoy with your morning coffee.

Ingredients

For the pumpkin bars:

- 1/3 cup organic pumpkin puree

- 1/3 cup coconut flour (sifted)

- 2 eggs (beaten)

- 2 tablespoons coconut oil

- 1/3 cup low-carb maple syrup

- 25 drops liquid sweetener of your choice

- 3 ½ tablespoons unsweetened coconut milk

- 2 teaspoons pumpkin pie spice

- 1 teaspoon sugar-free vanilla extract

- 1 teaspoon cinnamon

- 1 teaspoon apple cider vinegar

- ½ teaspoon baking soda

- 1/8 teaspoon sea salt

For the crumble topping:

- 1/3 cup raw almonds

- 3 tablespoons unsweetened flaked coconut

- 2 ½ tablespoons coconut oil (melted)

- 1 tablespoon granulated sugar substitute of your choice

- ¼ teaspoon cinnamon

Instructions

Grease an 8x8 baking dish or glass pan and set to the side. Set the oven to 350 degrees so it can preheat.

Put the coconut flour, pumpkin pie spice, cinnamon, and sea salt into a large bowl. Mix so all the ingredients are incorporated and set to the side. In another large bowl, add the pumpkin puree, eggs, coconut milk, sweetener, melted coconut oil, syrup, and vanilla extract. Whisk this together and set to the side.

In a small bowl, combine the baking soda and vinegar. This is going to bubble. Once the bubbles reduce, stir the baking soda mixture into the pumpkin-egg mixture until thoroughly incorporated. Then, stir the flour mixture in this bowl until all the ingredients are well combined. Spread this batter into the prepared baking dish and set to the side.

Next, add all the ingredients for the crumble to a mixing bowl. Mix the topping with a fork until it develops a paste-like consistency. Scatter chunks of this mixture across the top of

Pumpkin Crumble Bars

the pumpkin layer that is already in the baking dish. Cook for 28-30 minutes until you can insert a toothpick in the center of the bars and it comes out clean. The topping should be browned.

Once you remove the bars from the oven, allow to cool and then refrigerate at least one hour before serving so the pumpkin can set. Cut this into 9 bars.

Cast Iron Skillet Brownies with Peanut Butter Drizzle

These crispy-around-the-outside-and-gooey-in-the-middle brownies are just sweet enough to satisfy your sugar craving, but not so much that the flavors of the cocoa, vanilla, and nuts do not peek through. Additionally, there is only 12 grams of carbs in the entire 6" skillet full of brownie. This means that you can enjoy a guilt-free treat regardless of how many people you share it with.

Ingredients

For the brownies:

- 1 egg

- ¼ cup almond flour

- 6 tablespoons butter

- 1/3 cup cocoa powder

- 1/3 cup granulated sugar substitute of your choice

- ¼ cup walnuts (crushed to your preferred size)

- ½ teaspoon baking powder

- ½ teaspoon vanilla extract

- 1/8 teaspoon salt

Cast Iron Skillet Brownies with Peanut Butter Drizzle

For the peanut butter drizzle:

- 1 tablespoon butter

- 1 tablespoon peanut butter

Instructions

Set the oven to 350 degrees so it can preheat. Then, add the butter to a small saucepan and melt it over medium heat. Add the granulated sugar substitute and dissolve for about 5 minutes, until thoroughly incorporated. Transfer this to a medium-sized mixing bowl.

In the same bowl as the butter-sugar mixture, add the vanilla extract, cocoa powder, and salt. Mix this in and then add the egg. Beat the mixture until well combined and then incorporate the almond flower and baking powder. Finally, fold in the nuts and stir to combine.

Take the prepared brownie batter and pour it into a cast iron skillet, preferably a 6" skillet (for this recommended cooking time). Put this in the oven and cook for 30 minutes. The top of the brownie should be slightly jiggly, but still set. Remember that cast iron skillets retain heat and that your brownie will continue cooking once you remove it from the oven and be sure not to over-cook.

Just before the brownies are ready to come out of the oven, melt the butter and peanut butter in a small saucepan over medium heat. Once well-blended, pull off the heat and set to the side. You will drizzle this on your brownies once they start to cool.

Remember as you remove the skillet from the oven that the handle will be very hot and it will remain that way for a while. Use caution. If you drizzle the peanut butter topping on while the brownie is still warm, it will sink in more. If you drizzle it once the brownie has cooled, it will have a nicer presentation.

Easy Raspberry Linzer Cookie Bars

A traditional Linzer cookie requires a lot of rolling, layering, and in general, work. This recipe, by contrast, is a lot easier. It also has all the delicious flavors of a shortbread cookie with barely any carbs.

Ingredients

For the filling:

- ½ cup sugar-free raspberry preserves (with fiber)

- ¼ teaspoon almond extract

- ¼ teaspoon xanthan gum

For the crust:

- 2 cups almond flour

- ½ cup granulated sugar substitute of your choice

- 6 tablespoons butter (melted)

- ½ teaspoon sugar-free vanilla extract

Instructions

Start by preheating the oven to 350 degrees so it can preheat. Then, you are going to prepare the crust. Add all the ingredients for the crust to a medium bowl. Stir or mix with your hands to combine. This should result in a stiff dough. Set this to the side.

Next, you will prepare the filling. Combine the ingredients for the raspberry filling and stir until all are well incorporated.

When you are ready to assemble the cookie bars, layer a piece of parchment paper across an 8x8 baking pan. Press 2/3 of the crust mixture into the bottom. Place jelly mixture on top of this and use a spatula to spread. Then, take the remaining crust you have left and make a 'crumble' by placing chunks on top of the jelly.

Bake the prepared bars for 30 minutes. They should be firm and golden brown when they are done. Cool completely and cut the bars into 2-inch squares before enjoying.

Peanut Butter Cookies

Three ingredients are all it takes to throw together these delicious cookies. This is definitely a classic that you will keep on hand for your sweet tooth. They work as a before-bed snack with a glass of milk or even in the morning with a mug of coffee.

Ingredients

- 1 egg

- 1 cup peanut butter

- ½ cup powdered sugar substitute of your choice

Instructions

Set the oven to 350 degrees so it can preheat. Add all the ingredients to a medium mixing bowl and stir to combine. When you have a cookie dough consistency, roll these into 1-inch balls. Place these on a baking tray that has been lined with parchment paper.

Take a fork and press into each cookie twice, forming a 'criss cross' pattern on the top of the cookie. Bake for 10-15 minutes, until the edges start to get brown. Be cautious not to cook these too long- remember that they will firm up a little after they have been removed from the oven. Place them on a wire rack to cool to prevent overcooking and then enjoy!

Gingerbread Men Cookies

Who doesn't love decorating Gingerbread men- especially around the holiday season?

This low-carb cookie makes a great homemade gift, especially if you make them with the recommended low-carb icing. Just don't forget to be selective about how much candy you add.

This recipe makes about 40 4-inch gingerbread men.

Ingredients

For the cookies:

- 4 cups almond flour
- ¼ cup coconut flour
- 1 cup granulated sugar substitute of your choice
- ¼ cup coconut oil (melted)
- 2 large eggs
- 3 tablespoons molasses
- 2 teaspoons baking powder
- 3 tablespoons ground ginger

Savory Double Chocolate Macaroons

- 1 tablespoon cinnamon

- 1 teaspoon xanthan gum

- 1 teaspoon vanilla extract

- ½ teaspoon ground cloves

- ½ teaspoon salt

For the icing:

- ½ pound powdered sugar substitute of your choice

- ¼ cup slightly warm water (more as needed for thinning)

- 1 ½ tablespoons meringue powder

- 1/8 teaspoon xanthan gum

Instructions

Preheat the oven to 275 degrees.

If you want crispy gingerbread cookies instead of soft ones, preheat the oven to 225 degrees and bake for 50-60 minutes instead of following the directions later in this recipe.

Prepare two baking sheets by lining them with parchment paper and set them to the side.

Next, whisk together the dry cookie ingredients in a large bowl until they are all well-incorporated.

In a separate bowl, combine all the wet ingredients and mix well. Pour these into the dry ingredients and combine until a dough starts to form.

Take half the dough and place it between two sheets of parchment paper.

Use a rolling pin to flatten the dough until it is ¼ inch thick. Use cookie cutters to make the gingerbread men (you can also use other shapes).

Once you are done, continue to roll out the scraps and make men until you cannot.

Then, repeat with the remaining dough you set aside.

Place all the cookies on the wax paper-lined baking trays and cook for 20 minutes in the oven.

They should be slightly firm to the touch and golden brown in color.

Let these cool for 5 minutes before you remove them to cool completely on a wire rack.

While the cookies are cooling, create the frosting.

Mix the meringue powder, xanthan gum, and powdered sweetener in a bowl.

Add the warm water and mix until smooth.

Savory Double Chocolate Macaroons

You can add more water in 1 teaspoon increments until your icing is the right consistency.

Use these to decorate and add a few candies if you choose.

Savory Double Chocolate Macaroons

Dark chocolate, cinnamon, and a little bit of cinnamon powder give this savory macaroon incredible flavor. You can make these to enjoy yourself or give them as gifts to others. This is because the presentation is beautiful once you dip the macaroon in its coating.

Ingredients

- 2 cups unsweetened coconut (shredded)

- 2 large egg whites

- 1.8 ounces 90% dark chocolate

- 10-20 drops liquid artificial sweetener (optional)

- 1/3 cup unsweetened cocoa powder

- 1/3 cup coconut oil (melted)

- ¼ cup powdered sugar substitute of your choice

- 2 teaspoons cinnamon

- 1 teaspoon sugar-free vanilla extract

- ¼ teaspoon cayenne paper

- ¼ teaspoon sea salt

Savory Double Chocolate Macaroons

Instructions

Start by setting the oven to 350 degrees so it can preheat. Then, add the powdered sugar substitute, almond flour, shredded coconut, cacao powder, and dry seasonings to a large bowl and mix to thoroughly incorporate them all. Then, add the egg whites, vanilla extract, coconut oil, and liquid sweetener if you choose and mix to combine.

Next, line a baking sheet with parchment paper. Use a small ice cream scoop or a rounded measuring tablespoon to create round half-circle macaroons. Place these on the baking sheet and cook for 10-12 minutes in the oven.

While you are waiting for the macaroons to bake, prepare the chocolate dipping mixture. Melt the dark chocolate in a double boiler over medium heat. Remove it from the heat once melted completely and allow to cool, but do not allow it to solidify. You can re-warm if needed.

When the macaroons are baked, allow them to cool completely and then dip the tops into the chocolate one at a time. Lay the macaroons back on the parchment paper. If you choose, you can sprinkle additional cinnamon across the top. Let the chocolate solidify before eating- these can be stored at room temperature if you do not eat them all.

Section III:
Pies, Cakes, and Cheesecakes

Brownie Cheesecake

This chocolatey brownie crust and vanilla cheesecake topping pair deliciously together. This dessert is so sweet that it is almost sinful, but it is low-carb and gluten-free with less than 5 net carbs per serving. You will need a 9" springform pan to cook your cheesecake.

Ingredients

For the brownie crust:

- ¾ cup of granulated artificial sweetener (your preferred brand)

- 2 eggs

- ½ cup almond flour

- 2 ounces unsweetened chocolate (chopped)

- ¼ cup cocoa powder

- ½ cup butter (plus more for coating the pan)

- ¼ cup walnuts (chopped)

- ¼ teaspoon vanilla

- 1/8 teaspoon salt

For the cheesecake filling:

- 2 large eggs

- ¼ cup heavy cream

- 1 pound cream cheese (softened)

- ½ cup granulated artificial sweetener

- ½ teaspoon vanilla extract

Instructions

Start by buttering the springform pan. Wrap the bottom in foil and set to the side. Then, preheat the oven to 325 degrees.

Add the chopped chocolate and butter to a glass measuring cup or a microwave-safe bowl and microwave for 30 seconds at a time, until melted. Whisk the mixture together until it is smooth. Set this to the side.

Add the cocoa powder, almond flour, and salt to a small bowl and mix until combined. In a separate bowl (a large one), add the granulated sugar, eggs, and vanilla extract. Mix these together until smooth and then stir in the almond flour.

Once the brownie mixture is well-combined, stir in the butter/chocolate mixture until thoroughly incorporated. Then, stir in the chopped walnuts.

Spread the brownie mixture across the bottom of the springform pan and place in the preheated oven for 15 to 20 minutes. The mixture should still be soft in the center but the edges should be set. Set this to the side to cool for at least 15 to 20 minutes before topping with the cheesecake mixture.

While you are waiting for the crust to cool, you can prepare the filling. Reduce the oven temperature to 300 degrees so it can preheat.

Brownie Cheesecake

Then, add the cream cheese to a large bowl and use an electric mixer to beat until smooth. Then, stir in the eggs, heavy cream, granulated sugar substitute, and vanilla extract. When smooth and well combined, you are ready for the next step.

Place the springform pan on a baking sheet. Then, pour the cheesecake topping onto the prepared crust and bake for 35-45 minutes. The middle should jiggle barely and the edges should be set.

Let the cheesecake cool before taking a knife and using it to loosen the cheesecake. Remove the sides of the pan and then cover with plastic wrap. Refrigerate at least 3 hours before serving. You can top with a ganache or sugar-free chocolate sauce.

Pumpkin Cheesecake Tarts

These delicious tarts pair all the creaminess of a cheesecake with the sweet-and-spicy flavor of a pumpkin pie. They come together in a convenient little crust that you can pop in your mouth. This recipe makes 8 servings and should be prepared in 4 mini tartlet pans that are 4.5 inches in diameter.

Ingredients

For the filling:

- 1 cup pumpkin puree

- 1 cup ricotta cheese

- ¼ cup granulated sugar substitute of choice

- 2 eggs + 2 egg whites

- 2 teaspoons cinnamon

- 1 teaspoon vanilla extract

- ½ teaspoon pumpkin pie spice

- ¼ teaspoon salt

For the crust:

- 4 tablespoons butter (melted)

- 1 cup almond flour

- 2 teaspoons salt

- 1 pinch cinnamon

For the topping:

- 32 pecans

- Sugar-free maple syrup

Instructions

Start by preheating the oven to 350 degrees. You are going to make the crust first. Combine all the ingredients for the crust in a mixing bowl and mix until they are well combined. Press the resulting dough in the tartlet pans and place them in the oven for 10 minutes to prebake. Set to the side to cool once they are done so you can prepare the filling.

Add the pumpkin filling, ricotta cheese, eggs, and egg whites to a bowl and beat until they are well-combined. Then, add the remaining ingredients and mix until the seasonings are distributed throughout. If the crusts are cool, you can add these to the tart pans. These will not rise much, so you can fill the pans as high as you would like. Place these on a baking sheet and cook for about 20 minutes.

After 20 minutes, arrange the pecans in a circle on top of the tarts. Return to the oven for about 10 minutes. Allow to cool slightly and drizzle with the sugar-free maple syrup before serving.

Lava Cake

Moist cake and molten chocolate lava come together in this dish that will satisfy even the most intense chocolate cravings. You can enjoy the entire cake in this recipe for just 4 grams of carbohydrates. If you want a prettier presentation, you can dust some powdered sugar substitute on the top.

Ingredients

- 1 medium egg

- 2 tablespoons cocoa powder

- 2 tablespoons granulated sugar substitute of your choice

- 1 tablespoon heavy cream

- ½ teaspoon sugar-free vanilla extract

- ¼ teaspoon baking powder

- 1/8 teaspoon salt

Preheat the oven to 350 degrees. Place the cocoa powder and sugar substitute in a medium mixing bowl and whisk together until there are no clumps. In a separate bowl, beat the egg until it starts to become fluffy.

Add the beaten egg, vanilla extract, baking powder, heavy cream, and salt to the mixture. Stir until everything is well-combined. Then, spray a ramekin or ceramic mug with cooking oil. Cook it in the prepared oven for 10-15 minutes,

Lava Cake

being careful not to overcook. The top of the cake should be very jiggly, but set when it is done.

Pumpkin Spice Cake with Brown Butter Glaze

Savory pumpkin and sweet brown butter frosting come together in this recipe. It serves 12, with 7 grams of net carbs per serving. Be sure to set the pumpkin puree on a paper towel to sop up some extra moisture before you start cooking. This will stop your cake from becoming too gummy in texture.

Ingredients

For the cake:

- 2 cups almond flour

- 1 ½ cups pumpkin puree

- ½ cup granulated sugar substitute of your choice

- 1/3 cup whey protein powder (unflavored)

- 1/3 cup coconut flour

- 3 large eggs

- ¼ cup butter

- ¼ cup almond milk

- 1 tablespoon baking powder

- 2 teaspoons cinnamon

- 1 teaspoon vanilla extract

- 1 teaspoon ginger

- ½ teaspoon liquid artificial sweetener of your choice

- ½ teaspoon cloves

For the glaze:

- 2 cups powdered sugar substitute of your choice (sifted)

- ½ cup butter (softened)

- ¼ cup cream (room temperature)

Instructions

Place two layers of a strong paper towel on a plate and spread the pumpkin puree across it. Add an additional 2 layers on top of the mixture and allow to sit for 20 minutes. While you are waiting, coat 2 8-inch round cake pans with coconut oil or butter. Layer a piece of parchment paper across the bottom of each and grease this as well.

Then, set the oven to 325 degrees to preheat. Whisk together the coconut and almond flours, protein powder, baking powder, and spices in a bowl to combine. Set this to the side.

Add the dried pumpkin puree, butter, and sugar substitute to a large bowl and beat until they have a smooth consistency. Then, beat in the eggs, liquid sweetener, and vanilla extract. Add half the almond flour mixture and half the almond milk and beat thoroughly. Then, repeat with the remaining almond flour and milk. You should have a thick batter. If it is stiff and hard to mix, add another tablespoon of almond milk at a time until it is easier to beat.

Put half the prepared batter in each of the greased cake pans and use a spatula to smooth the top. Bake until you can insert a toothpick in the center and it comes out clean. The edges of the cake will be browned. This should take about 40 minutes. Let the cakes cool inside the pan for about 20 minutes before turning upside down on a wire rack and removing the pan.

While you are waiting, prepare the brown butter glaze. Add the butter to a saucepan and cook over a medium flame. You want to continue cooking until the butter becomes fragrant and brown. Add the powdered sweetener to a bowl and then add the browned butter, beating until well combined. Then, add the cream and beat until the icing is a spreadable consistency.

Once the cakes have completely cooled, you can ice them. Place one cake on a serving platter and cover with icing and repeat with the second, placing it on top of the first.

Irish Cream Cheesecake

Hints of coffee and Irish cream make this cheesecake unique. It remains light, fluffy, and easy to make. Even being a cheesecake, you do not have to bake this. You can layer it into a large pan or fill up a few small bowls. This recipe makes 8 servings.

Ingredients

For the filling:

- 8 ounces cream cheese (softened)

- 1 cup heavy whipping cream

- ½ cup low-carb Irish cream

- 1/3 cup granulated sugar substitute of your choice

- 3 tablespoons cocoa (unsweetened)

- 3 tablespoons butter (softened)

- 2 tablespoons powdered sugar substitute of your choice

- 2 teaspoons sugar-free vanilla extract

- 2 teaspoons hot water

- 2 teaspoons cold water

- 1 teaspoon gelatin

For the crust:

- ¾ cup almond flour

- 3 tablespoons butter (melted)

- 2 ½ tablespoons cocoa

- 2 tablespoons granulated sugar substitute of your choice

Instructions

You are going to prepare the crust first. Combine the dry ingredients first and mix to incorporate. Then, add the melted butter and mix until you have a crust-like consistency. Press this into a large pan or 8 dessert cups.

Then, you will prepare the filling. Add the butter and cream cheese to a large mixing bowl and beat with an electric mixture to combine. Then, mix in the Irish cream, granulated sweetener, cocoa, and vanilla extract until smooth. Set this to the side.

Add the whipping cream to another mixing bowl and add the powdered sweetener. Whip until soft peaks start to form. Set this to the side.

Add the cold water to a small cup. Sprinkle the gelatin on top and allow to sit until it becomes soft. Then, add the hot water and stir the mixture until the gelatin has dissolved completely.

Begin whipping the sweetened heavy cream again and gradually add the gelatin. Whip until stiff peaks form. Then, gently fold this mixture into the Irish cream mixture that was set to the side.

Irish Cream Cheesecake

Place this on top of the crust and use a spatula to smooth the top.

Then, transfer to the refrigerator and allow to chill for at least 2 hours before enjoying.

Chocolate French Silk Pie

This spin on a classic comes with the smooth, creamy texture and all the flavors of French silk pie. It also comes with a lot less carbs and a melt-in-your-mouth peanut butter crust.

Ingredients

For the chocolate filling:

- 4 ounces unsweetened baker's chocolate (melted)

- 1/3 cup + 1/3 cup powdered sugar substitute of your choice

- 3 large eggs

- ¾ cup unsalted butter (salted)

- 1 tablespoon vanilla extract

- ¼ teaspoon salt

For the crust:

- 1 cup peanut flour

- 1 large egg

- ¼ cup almond milk

- 2 tablespoons protein powder

- 2 tablespoons powdered sugar substitute

- 1 tablespoon coconut oil (melted)

- ½ teaspoon sea salt

For the topping:

- 1 cup heavy cream

- 1 tablespoon powdered sugar substitute

- Chocolate shavings (optional for garnish)

Instructions

You are going to make your crust first. Start by preheating the oven to 350 degrees. Add the peanut flour, sea salt, protein powder, and sugar substitute to a large bowl and mix to combine. Then, add the wet ingredients and stir. You may want to use your hands- the result should be a sticky, dough-like mixture. Press this into a 9" pie pan. When you are done, pierce the bottom with a fork so it does not bubble while cooking. Put the prepared pie crust in the oven for about 8-10 minutes, until golden brown in color.

Next, you will prepare the chocolate silk filling. Place the eggs and 1/3 cup of the sugar substitute in a double boiler. Whisk them together over the heat for about 5-10 minutes. The sugar should dissolve completely and the eggs should be thick and pale. Take them off the stove and allow them to cool while you prepare the rest of the mix.

Add the remaining sugar and the butter to a bowl and mix with an electric beater until well-combined. Then, beat in the melted chocolate, salt, and vanilla extract. Once everything is blended in, add the cooling egg mixture and stir until everything is incorporated. Once your crust is completely cooled, add this to the pie pan.

Finally, you will prepare the whipped topping. Add the heavy whipping cream and the sugar substitute to a bowl and beat until you have about three times as much as you started with and the mixture is thick. Top your pie with the whipped topping and garnish with chocolate shavings.

Personal Red Velvet Cinnamon Cheesecake

This cheesecake features a cinnamon-y cheesecake layer atop a rich, red velvet crust. Aside from the rich and savory flavors, you can eat an entire mini cheesecake for just 2 grams of carbohydrates.

Ingredients

For the red velvet layer:

- 1 egg

- 1/3 cup powdered sugar substitute of your choice

- ¼ cup butter

- 6 tablespoons almond flour

- 1 tablespoon cocoa powder

- 1 teaspoon red food coloring

- ½ teaspoon apple cider vinegar

- ½ teaspoon sugar-free vanilla extract

- 1/8 teaspoon salt

For the cheesecake layer:

- 1 egg

- 6 ounces cream cheese (softened)

- 2 tablespoons powdered sugar substitute of your choice

- 1 tablespoon butter (softened)

- 1 teaspoon cinnamon

- ½ teaspoon sugar-free vanilla extract

- 1/8 teaspoon salt

Instructions

You are going to prepare the red velvet layer of the cake first. Begin by setting the oven to 350 degrees so it can preheat. Then, add the butter to a small sauce pan and warm over low heat. Once it is melted, stir in the powdered sugar and continue to cook over low heat, stirring periodically, until the sugar is completely dissolved.

Add the butter-sugar mixture to a large bowl and combine it with the vanilla, cocoa powder, and salt. Add the egg and mix until all the ingredients are thoroughly incorporated. Then, add the apple cider vinegar and food coloring. Once these are stirred in, add the almond flour and mix until combined. Set to the side for a moment.

Grease 4 small ramekins and then pour the red velvet mixture inside. Lightly tap the side a few times, until the top of the batter starts to even out and all the air bubbles have been released. Place the ramekins on a baking tray and set them inside the refrigerator as you prepare the next layer.

Add the butter and cream cheese to a bowl. Beat this mixture with an electric mixer until it develops a light and fluffy texture. Then, beat in the egg, cinnamon, and vanilla extract. Finally, add the powdered sweetener and salt and beat one more time, until all the ingredients are distributed throughout.

Personal Red Velvet Cinnamon Cheesecake

Remove the ramekins from the refrigerator and add 2 heaping tablespoons of the cheesecake mixture on each. Place these in the oven for about 20 minutes. You will know they are done when the cheesecake is jiggly, but set on top. Let them cool for a while before eating. For a more cheesecake-like experience, refrigerate a few hours before enjoying. Otherwise, you can enjoy this warm.

Chocolate Iced Donuts

This recipe contains protein powder, so you might expect that these would be dense or cardboard-like in texture. Instead, the process used to make these makes them light and fluffy. The secret is in the way you whip the egg whites and fold in the ingredients- follow the instructions closely or they will not turn out fluffy. You can top with chopped walnuts or pecans if you want a little crunch. Also, you will need a donut pan to make these.

Ingredients

For the icing:

- 2 tablespoons heavy cream

- 2 scoops 100% Casein chocolate protein powder (you can use a different flavor if you do not want chocolate icing)

For the donut:

- 3 eggs (separated)

- ½ cup ground almonds

- ½ cup granulated low-calorie sweetener of your choice

- 2 tablespoons melted butter

- 2 tablespoons pure cocoa powder

- 1 teaspoon vanilla extract

Personal Red Velvet Cinnamon Cheesecake

- ¼ teaspoon baking powder

- ¼ teaspoon cinnamon

- ¼ teaspoon salt

Instructions

Start by preheating your oven to 350 degrees while you prepare the donuts. Take the egg whites and whip them in a bowl. You will need to mix them a lot, so you may want to use a mixer. Whip them until the whites have stiff peaks.

In a separate bowl, mix the dry ingredients for the donuts until they are well combined. Then, add the egg yolks, butter, and granulated artificial sugar to a third bowl and whisk together until all the ingredients are thoroughly incorporated.

Next, use extreme caution to gently fold the sugar, egg yolk, and butter mixture into the egg whites. Then, slowly add the dry ingredients and mix gently to combine. Be careful not to over-mix.

Fill each of the molds in the donut pan until they are ¾ of the way full. Bake for about 15 minutes, until you can insert a toothpick for the donuts and they come out clean.

To prepare the frosting, whip together the heavy cream and casein powder until the frosting becomes thick. You can let the donuts cool and then frost them, or you can use the frosting as a dipping sauce and enjoy them right out of the oven.

Chocolate Cheesecake

Who doesn't love a good cheesecake? The texture of this cheesecake is creamy and it has just enough sweetness to satisfy your craving. The crust and the filling are both made of chocolate. You will need a springform pan to make this cheesecake.

Ingredients

For the filling:

- 16 ounces cream cheese (softened)

- 3 ounces unsweetened baker's chocolate

- ¾ cup powdered sugar substitute of choice

- ½ cup sour cream

- 2 eggs

- 1 tablespoon cocoa powder

- 1 teaspoon vanilla extract

- 1/8 teaspoon salt

For the crust:

- 4 tablespoons butter

- 1 cup almond flour

- 1 tablespoon cocoa powder

Chocolate Cheesecake

- Few drops of liquid sweetener to taste

- ½ teaspoon cinnamon

- 1/8 teaspoon salt

Instructions

Start by setting the oven to 350 degrees so it can preheat. You are going to make the crust first. Add everything except the butter and liquid sweetener to the bowl. Mix these to combine. Melt the butter. Just before you add it to the dry ingredients for the crust, add a few drops of liquid sweetener. Mix until you have a dough-like consistency.

Press the crust into the bottom of the springform pan. Place this in the oven to cook for 15 minutes, until the crust forms a solid layer and becomes darker in color.

While you are waiting, you can prepare the chocolate cheesecake filling. Start by beating the powdered sugar and cream cheese together in a large bowl with an electric mixture until you have a smooth consistency. Then, add in the sour cream, eggs, vanilla extract, and salt. Continue to beat until the cheesecake becomes smooth and creamy. Set this to the side.

Melt the baker's chocolate in a double boiler. Once melted, stir this and the cocoa powder into the cream cheese filling. Pour this on top of the crust and place in the oven. Cook for 50-60 minutes.

You will know it is done when the cheesecake has become darker and sets on the top. The underside will still be slightly jiggly.

Allow this to cool. Once the cheesecake reaches room temperature, place it in the refrigerator to cool. It would be ideal to let it cool overnight so the cheesecake firms, but a few hours will suffice.

Then, use a knife along the edge of the springform pan and remove the sides. Cut into 8 pieces.

Lemon Meringue Tarts

Who doesn't love fluffy meringue and tart lemon? These tarts have all the flavor of lemon meringue pie in a smaller morsel. This recipe makes 4 tarts that are 4.5" in diameter, with 2 servings in each tart.

Ingredients

For the crust:

- 2 cups almond flour

- 4 tablespoons powdered sugar substitute of your choice

- 4 tablespoons whey protein

- 1 egg

- 2 tablespoons butter

- 1/2 teaspoon salt

For the lemon curd:

- 6 egg yolks

- 1/2 cup powdered sugar substitute

- 1/2 cup butter

- 4 lemons

- 20 drops liquid sweetener

- 1/4 teaspoon xanthan gum

For the meringue:

- 4 tablespoons powdered sweetener

- 4 egg whites

- 1/4 teaspoon cream of tartar

Instructions

Start by setting the oven to 350 degrees to preheat. Then, you will make the crust. Combine all the ingredients in a bowl and mix with your hands. When you have a dough ball, press it into 4 separate tart pans. Cook these for 12-15 minutes, checking frequently to make sure it does not burn.

While you are waiting, zest 2 of your lemons. In the same bowl, add the juice of all 4 lemons. Set this to the side.

In a separate bowl, add the egg yolks and whisk them with the liquid sweetener and powdered sugar substitute. Once well combined, pour these into a double boiler and continue to whisk. Cook for 10 minutes, until the substance becomes thick. Then, pour in the lemon zest and juice combination that you set aside. Continue to whisk until the entire solution is warmed through.

Then, add the xanthan gum to thicken the solution. Break up the butter into small parts, whisking in one piece at a time until it is melted and completely combined. When all the butter is added, turn off the heat and refrigerate the lemon curd until you are ready to assemble the tarts.

Lemon Meringue Tarts

Next, you will prepare the meringue. Put the egg whites in a bowl and use an electric mixer to beat them on low speed until they have a frothy consistency. This should take about 5 minutes. Continue whipping as you add the cream of tartar. Then, add 1 tablespoon of the powdered sweetener at a time as you turn up the beater to medium speed. Once all the sweetener has been added, whip on high speed until stiff peaks start to form in the egg whites. This will take about 5 more minutes.

Now, assemble the tarts. Divide the lemon curd evenly among the 4 tartlets and top with the meringue. Bake at 325 degrees for 12 minutes, until the peaks of the meringue have become golden.

Section IV: Frozen Desserts

Strawberry Basil Icy Bites

This recipe combines fresh strawberry and basil, which is great since these things are in season around the same time. It is cool and refreshing. You can easily pop one out of the freezer and into your mouth whenever you want for a delicious icy treat. You will need a silicone muffin mold to make these bites- this recipe makes 10.

Ingredients

- ¾ + ¼ cup fresh strawberries (cleaned and de-stemmed)

- 2 tablespoons fresh basil

- ¾ cup cream cheese

- ½ cup creamed coconut milk (room temperature)

- ¼ coconut oil

- ¼ cup powdered sugar substitute of your choice

- 1 teaspoon sugar-free

- Liquid sweetener to taste (optional)

Instructions

Add the cream cheese, creamed coconut milk, sugar, vanilla extract, and coconut oil to a food processor and pulse until it is a smooth and creamy texture. Taste it and add liquid sweetener if you want. If so, add the sweetener and pulse again to incorporate.

Take half of the prepared mixture and set it to the side. Leave the other half in the processor and add the ¾ cup of strawberries. Blend until smooth. Then, divide the mixture evenly in the muffin molds.

Wash out the food processor and put the cream cheese mixture you set to the side inside it. Then, add the basil and pulse the mixture until it is smooth. Add 1 ½ tablespoons of this on top of the strawberry cream cheese mixture you already placed in the molds. Then, take the remaining ¼ cup of strawberry and cut them into slices. Top each of your bites with a few of these slices and freeze 2-3 hours before enjoying.

Protein Powder Ice Cream

This protein-packed dessert is cool and refreshing. You can make it with your preferred flavor and then top with low-carb fruits like raspberries or blueberries. It is also super simple to make, needing just two ingredients.

Ingredients

- 3 tablespoons heavy whipping cream

- 1 scoop Whey Protein powder

Instructions

Add the two ingredients to a medium bowl. Mix them together, either with a whisk or using a hand blender until the cream thickens. Cover and place in the freezer for at least an hour before serving. You want it to be frozen.

Strawberry Pistachio Dreamsicles

Sweet strawberries and salty pistachios come together in this frozen treat. They pair well with a creamy background that is every bit as good as a sugar-filled dreamsicle.

Ingredients

- 8 ounces strawberries (cleaned with stems removed)

- 2 ounces salted pistachios (without shells)

- ½ cup almond milk

- ½ cup heavy cream

- Liquid artificial sweetener to taste

Instructions

Add all the ingredients except the pistachios to the food processor. Blend until the mixture is smooth and creamy. Then, continue to blend for a minute so that the mixture start to aerate and become fluffy.

Add the pistachios in and stir with a spoon to distribute throughout. Pour this into popsicle molds and place in the freezer for at least 2 hours, or until set completely.

Tiramisu Ice Cream Bites

The delicious flavors of tiramisu and the texture of smooth, creamy ice cream come together in this bite that you can easily pop in your mouth. The creamy, cool flavors of tiramisu ice cream is coated in melt-in-your-mouth dark chocolate. You can make these in candy molds, silicone muffin molds, or cake pop molds.

For the chocolate coating:

- 1 ounce cacao butter

- 1.4 ounces 90% dark chocolate

For the tiramisu ice cream filling:

- 1 ¼ cups full-fat mascarpone cheese

- ¼ cup chilled brewed coffee (with a strong flavor)

- ¼ cup powdered sugar substitute of your choice

- 1 ½ teaspoons sugar-free rum extract

- Liquid sweetener to taste

Instructions

Combine the mascarpone, powdered sweetener, chilled coffee, and rum extract in a bowl with a mixer or in a food processor until creamy. Add sweetener to taste and briefly mix to incorporate.

Add about 2 tablespoons of this mixture into your molds. You should be able to make 12 ice cream bites. Place these in the freezer for at least 2 hours before starting the next step so they set.

Just before you are ready to coat the tiramisu balls, melt the cacao butter and chocolate using a double boiler. Mix them together until they are smooth and then allow the mixture to cool. It should remain liquid, but you do not want it to be so hot that it melts the ice cream balls.

As you coat the balls, it is important that you do not melt them. Remove 3-4 ice cream bombs from the freezer at a time. Before you start, line a baking sheet with parchment paper. You will place your ice cream balls on this.

Use a toothpick to poke one ball at a time. Hold this over the bowl of melted chocolate and use a tablespoon to pour the chocolate over it. Turn it so you coat the entire ball. If the chocolate is cool enough, it should solidify. Place the coated ice cream bombs in the freezer for at least 15 minutes before enjoying.

Dark Chocolate Ice Cream

There are not vanilla or other flavors peeking out of this ice cream. It is for the serious chocolate lover and it has a rich, dark chocolate taste that will satisfy. You will need an ice cream maker for this recipe.

- 2 cups heavy cream

- 4 large eggs

- 3 ounces unsweetened chocolate (chopped)

- ½ cup cocoa powder

- ½ cup granulated sugar substitute of your choice

- 1 cup + ½ cup unsweetened coconut milk

- ½ teaspoon vanilla extract

- ½ teaspoon liquid sweetener to taste

- 2 tablespoons vodka (optional, to reduce iciness)

Instructions

Place a large bowl in an ice bath and set to the side. Then, combine 1 cup of the cashew milk with the cream, cocoa powder, and your chosen sweetener. Whisk these together and then stir frequently until the cream mixture reaches a temperature of 170 degrees.

While you are waiting for the cream to come to temperature, whisk together the egg yolks in a bowl. Add about 1 cup of the hot cream mixture, continuously beating so the eggs reach temperature. Slowly whisk this back into the saucepan and continue to cook the mixture until it reaches 175 degrees and is thick enough to coat the backside of a spoon instead of dripping off.

Then, remove the pan from the heat and put the chopped chocolate in. Let this sit for 5 minutes before whisking together until smooth. Then, carefully pour the chocolate cream in the bowl that you placed in the ice bath. Let this cool for 10 minutes before covering in plastic. Place it in the refrigerator for three hours.

When your chocolate cream has chilled long enough, whisk in the remaining cashew milk, vanilla extract, and vodka. The mixture may be hard to stir at first, because it will be very thick. You will need to whisk vigorously to incorporate everything. Then, pour the mixture into the ice cream maker and prepare according to the instructions provided by the manufacturer. Once it is finished, you may enjoy right away as a soft serve or store in the freezer for 1-2 hours and enjoy as a firmer ice cream.

Strawberry Swirl Ice Cream

This ice cream has ribbons of sweet-yet-tart strawberries inside. You can either prepare it in an ice cream maker or freeze it in the freezer to help it firm up. The vodka is optional, but it will help cut back the iciness that you sometimes get with frozen desserts, especially those containing artificial sweeteners.

Ingredients

- 3 large egg yolks

- 1 cup heavy cream

- 1 cup strawberries (pureed, with a few chunks)

- 1/3 cup granulated sugar substitute of your choice

- 1 tablespoon vodka (optional)

- ½ teaspoon vanilla extract

Instructions

Gently warm the heavy cream in a saucepan using low heat. Do not allow it to simmer or boil. Once warm, add the sugar substitute and allow to warm until it dissolves completely. While you are waiting, add the yolks to a deep mixing bowl and beat with an electric mixer. Continue to beat until the egg mixture has doubled in size.

Then, slowly add a few tablespoons of the cream mixture at a time. This will temper the eggs, so they do not cook. Beat the eggs as you do this. Once the egg mixture is warm enough, add the remaining cream and continue to beat. Then, add the vanilla extract. Finally, beat in the vodka if you are choosing to use it.

Put the prepared ice cream mix in the freezer for 1-2 hours. You will need to stir it occasionally. Alternatively, you can use an ice cream mixer. Just follow the manufacturer's instructions.

Once your ice cream starts to firm, it is time to add in the strawberries. If you have not pureed them yet, do so now. You want some chunks, but the rest should be pureed. Stir this into your ice cream, incorporating it throughout. Be careful not to over-mix though. The key to strawberry swirl is ribbons of strawberry throughout white ice cream. Return to the freezer for 4-6 hours before serving.

Mint Chocolate Chip Ice Cream Bites

Who doesn't love mint chocolate chip ice cream? These tasty bites are made of avocado ice cream flavored with fresh mint and chunks of dark chocolate. You can freeze the bites in a cake pop mold if you want a round shape, but a silicone muffin mold will work as well. This recipe makes 8 bites.

Ingredients

- 1 cup full-fat mascarpone cheese

- Flesh of 1 medium ripe avocado

- 2 ounces 80-90% dark chocolate (chopped)

- ¼ cup + 1 tablespoon powdered sugar substitute of your choice

- 1 tablespoon fresh mint (chopped)

- Liquid sweetener to taste (optional)

Instructions

Add the mascarpone, avocado flesh, powdered sweetener, and mint to a food processor and pulse until you have a smooth consistency. Taste this and add the liquid sweetener if you would like. Pulse to combine. Then, add the dark chocolate and pulse to incorporate, being sure not to mix too long so you do not break the chocolate into tiny bits.

Use a tablespoon to place 2 tablespoons in each of your molds. Freeze for at least 2 hours before enjoying.

Section V:
Puddings, Mousses, and More

Quick Peanut Butter Mousse

This mousse is light, fluffy, and can be on the table in less than five minutes. Its aerated texture allows the rich peanut butter flavor to melt on your tongue. Top with dark chocolate shavings as a garnish if you would like. This recipe makes 3 servings at 4 grams of carbohydrates each.

Ingredients

- 1 cup heavy whipping cream

- 4 ounces cream cheese

- 1/3 cup liquid artificial sweetener (more or less to taste)

- 2 tablespoons no-sugar-added peanut butter

- ½ teaspoon sugar-free vanilla extract

Instructions

Add the heavy whipping cream to a medium bowl and mix it with an electric mixer until it firms up and has stiff peaks. Set this to the side.

Take a second medium bowl and combine all the remaining ingredients. Mix these together until you achieve a creamy, smooth texture and all the ingredients are incorporated. Taste this and decide if you need additional sweetener before continuing.

Then, add the whipped cream to the peanut butter mixture. Whip the entire mixture for about one minute, until there are no lumps and the mousse has developed a light and fluffy texture. Refrigerate or enjoy immediately.

Watermelon Cream Soup

Most Keto recipes contain berries, since those are low in carbs and high in fiber. Watermelon, however, is mostly made of water so it is safe to eat. The added fat from the sour cream makes this delicious and hearty (as well as Keto-approved).

Ingredients

- ¾ cup seeded watermelon chunks

- ¼ cup heavy cream

- ¼ cup raspberries

- 2 tablespoons sour cream

- 1 tablespoon vanilla artificial sweetener

- ¼ teaspoon fresh mint (chopped)

- ¼ teaspoon lemon juice

Instructions

Add all the ingredients except the heavy whipping cream to a blender. Pulse until the mixture is smooth. Pour this into a small bowl and refrigerate while you prepare the whipped topping.

Place the heavy cream in a bowl and beat with an electric mixer. If you choose, you can add a few drops of your favorite sweetener to give it a more authentic whipped cream taste. The cream should be stiff after a minute or so of beating.

Remove the watermelon soup from the fridge and top with the whipped cream.

Salted Caramel Panna Cotta

This plain panna cotta is creamy, sweet, and delicious. It offers beautiful mild flavors that can be paired with nearly any flavor. In this recipe, it is sweet caramel and salt that comes together for a sweet-and salty pairing that will tantalize your taste buds. Each of these 4 servings contains just 6 carbohydrates.

Ingredients

- 2 cups heavy cream

- 1 packet gelatin (unflavored)

- ½ cup caramel

- ¼ cup powdered sugar substitute of your choice

- 1 teaspoon sugar-free vanilla extract

- ½ teaspoon coarse sea salt

Instructions

Add the cream to a medium saucepan and place over low heat. Allow it to warm, being very careful not to bring to a simmer. Then, stir in the powdered sweetener and gelatin. Continue to warm until these are dissolved, whisking frequently. Once they are dissolved, add the vanilla extract. Set this to the side for a moment.

Grease 4 ramekins or ceramic dishes and then pour the panna cotta mixture inside. Allow these to chill at least 2 hours. Ideally, you will chill overnight before serving. When you are ready to enjoy, top each with ¼ of the caramel and a slight sprinkling of sea salt. You can enjoy straight from the ramekin or use a knife to loosen the edges and dump on a plate.

Mexican Chocolate Pudding

This pudding uses avocado as a base, with plenty of chocolate and a hint of spice from cayenne pepper and Ceylon cinnamon. Be sure to use Ceylon cinnamon and not Cassia cinnamon- this will make a big difference in the final taste of your pudding.

Ingredients

- 1 avocado

- 2 ½ tablespoons raw cocoa powder

- 1 tablespoon coconut milk

- 1 tablespoon liquid sweetener of your choice

- 1 teaspoon Ceylon cinnamon

- ½ teaspoon sugar-free vanilla extract

- 1/8 teaspoon sea salt

- 1/8 teaspoon sugar substitute of choice

- 1/16 teaspoon cayenne pepper

Instructions

Cut the avocado in half, remove the flesh, and scoop the flesh out with a spoon. Place this in a food processor or blender and puree until smooth. Place the coconut milk, cocoa powder, and vanilla extract in the processor as well and blend until well combined. Then, add the sweetener, sugar substitute, cinnamon, and cayenne pepper and pulse until combined.

Use a spoon to scrape any chunks down the side of the food processor and continue to blend. Repeat this process until all the mixture is smooth- this is the consistency that is necessary for pudding.

You can enjoy this right away or refrigerate for a few hours first. For a little crunch and a sweet-salty flavor combo, top with a sprinkle of the sea salt just before serving.

Lemon Panna Cotta with Raspberry Jam Topping

Tart lemon and sweet-but-tart raspberry come together in this creamy recipe. If you do not know what a panna cotta is- it is a jello-like dessert. However, it is a lot creamier than traditional gelatin and you will find this recipe is a lot more flavorful as well.

Ingredients

- 1 cup unsweetened almond milk

- 1 cup heavy cream

- 1 packet gelatin (unflavored)

- ½ cup sugar-free raspberry jam

- ¼ cup granulated sugar substitute of your choice

- 1 tablespoon fresh lemon juice

- 1 teaspoon sugar-free vanilla extract

- Raspberries for garnish (optional)

Instructions

Add the almond milk and heavy cream to a medium sauce pan and allow it to warm over a low flame. Then, stir in the gelatin and sugar substitute. Allow these to dissolve, but do not let this mixture come to a boil. Whisk constantly while you wait.

Once the ingredients are all incorporated, turn off the stove and add the lemon juice and vanilla extract. Set this to the side for a moment. Prepare 4 ramekins or other ceramic dishes by lightly spraying them with oil. Then, pour the panna cotta batter evenly among the dishes.

Cover each of these individually and allow to sit in the refrigerator for at least 2 hours. Ideally, you will leave them in the refrigerator overnight. When you are ready to serve the panna cotta, use a knife and run it along the edge of the ramekins. This will loosen the panna cotta. Turn the dishes upside down and onto a plate. Then, top with the sugar-free raspberry jelly and add a few fresh raspberries as a garnish.

Chia Pudding

This pudding is high in fiber because of the chia seeds and hemp hearts, both which can likely be found at your local health food store. Be sure to adhere to the guidelines about storing in the refrigerator at least overnight. Otherwise, the seeds will remain crunchy. This pudding can be enjoyed as a dessert anytime, but it is also so healthy that you could eat it as a filling breakfast.

Ingredients

- ¼ cup vanilla almond milk (unsweetened)

- 3 tablespoons chia seeds

- 2 tablespoons hemp hearts

- 1 tablespoon chopped almonds

- 1 tablespoon chopped pecans

- 1 tablespoon flaked coconut (unsweetened)

- 1 teaspoon pine nuts

Instructions

Add all the ingredients to a bowl and mix well. Once everything is incorporated, cover and put in the fridge overnight.

The chia seeds will swell and soften. If you find the mixture to be too dry the next morning, stir in a little almond milk at a time until the desired consistency is reached.

You can eat as is or top with sugar-free maple syrup, cinnamon, dark chocolate chips, or fresh or frozen fruit.

Chocolate Mascarpone Mousse

Rich, creamy mascarpone and dreamy chocolate come together in this recipe. It is aerated perfectly so that the mousse literally melts in your mouth. This recipe has less than 2 grams of net carbs per serving and can be made in under 5 minutes.

Ingredients

- 1 cup mascarpone cheese

- 2 tablespoons cocoa powder (unsweetened)

- 1 tablespoon heavy cream (or more if mousse becomes too thick)

- 1 tablespoon granulated sugar substitute of your choice

- 1 teaspoon sugar-free vanilla extract

Instructions

Add all the ingredients except the heavy cream to a medium bowl. Mix them well with an electric beater, mixing to aerate. If the mousse seems to heavy, add the heavy cream. You may also add another tablespoon, one at a time until the right consistency is reached. Taste and adjust the sweetness if needed and then place in glass bowls. This recipe makes 4 servings.

Conclusion

The decision to switch to a Ketogenic Diet can be a life-changing one, regardless of if you are trying to lose weight or trying to manage a medical condition. There are many benefits to this diet, especially when done the right way. Perhaps one of the best things about the Keto Diet is that you do not have to give up sweet or savory desserts, as you should see from reading through the recipes in this book.

The next logical step is to compile a list of groceries for some of the recipes you want to try and head to the store! Since many of these recipes (especially the candies) store well, you can easily make them in advance and keep them on hand. This means that you can have instant sweet tooth satisfaction whenever you may need it to keep you from giving into your cravings.

So, get your groceries and start cooking! You may be overwhelmed by the number of dessert recipes you want to try. Don't worry, you will have plenty of time to try all of them through the duration of your Ketogenic Diet.

Finally, if you enjoyed this book, then I'd like to ask you for a favor, would you be kind enough to leave a review for this book on Amazon? It'd be greatly appreciated!

Best of luck and happy eating!